COOKBOOK FOR CARNIVORES' DIET FOR BEGINNERS

"Savoring Simplicity: A Beginner's Guide to Carnivorous Cuisine"

ELENA GEORGE

Copyright © [2024] by [Elena George]

This book is a work of non-fiction. Names, characters, places, and incidents are either the product of the author's imagination or are used fictitiously. Any resemblance to actual persons, living or dead, events, or locales is entirely coincidental.

Table of contents

INTRODUCTION

Welcome to the world of carnivorous cuisine! This cookbook takes us on a delicious journey explicitly designed for beginners who want to explore the wonders of carnivore eating and dieting. Whether you are looking for better health and more energy or want to eat delicious meat dishes, you are at the right place.

The carnivore diet, characterized by the exclusion of plant foods and an emphasis on animal foods, has received considerable attention in recent years.

These pages delve into the basics of carnivore diets and provide the knowledge and skills you need to succeed on this unique culinary journey.

From understanding dietary principles to mastering basic cooking techniques, each chapter is designed to help you create mouth-watering dishes highlighting animal protein's richness and variety. You'll find many mouth-watering recipes, from hearty breakfasts to hearty dinners, delicious sides and appetizers, and even carnivore-friendly desserts.

Whether you're an experienced on the carnivore diet or you're a beginner to this way of eating, there's something to learn for everyone. But this cookbook is more than just a collection of recipes.

A guide to living a lifestyle based on healthy, nutritious food that nourishes your body and mind.

As you read along, we'll share practical tips for planning meals, buying quality ingredients, and confidently handling social situations.

So, make this cookbook your trusted companion in your culinary adventures, whether you're ready to engage in the carnivore lifestyle or simply looking to incorporate more Animal protein into your diet. Get ready to taste the flavors, get creative in the kitchen, and discover the joy of eating proteinous animal cuisines. Let's start!

CHAPTER ONE

What is the Carnivore Diet?

A carnivore diet is a dietary approach that excludes plant foods and favors the consumption of animal products. This restrictive diet typically includes meat, fish, eggs, and other animal products, with minimal or no intake of fruits, vegetables, grains, legumes, or other plant food. The core of the carnivore diet is based on the belief that animal foods are the most nutritious and bioavailable source of essential nutrients such as protein, fat, vitamins, and minerals. Proponents of this diet believe that eliminating plant foods containing antinutrients and other compounds complex for some people to digest and tolerate improves health, digestion, and various health benefits. It is claimed that the above problem can be alleviated. The carnivore diet is considered an extreme or unconventional approach to nutrition because it departs from traditional dietary principles that promote a balanced intake of plant and animal foods. However, proponents of this diet say it can offer many potential benefits, including weight loss, improved metabolic health, increased mental clarity, and reduced inflammation. It's important to note that the carnivore diet is unsuitable for everyone, and its long-term health effects have not been well studied. Critics of this diet have expressed concerns about its nutritional adequacy, potential risk of dietary deficiencies, and lack of scientific evidence supporting its long-term effectiveness and safety. Ultimately, whether a carnivore diet is suitable for an individual depends on a variety of factors, including the individual's health status, dietary preferences, and personal beliefs. As with any dietary approach, it's essential to consult a medical professional or nutritionist before making any significant changes to your diet, especially if it's as restrictive as a carnivore diet.

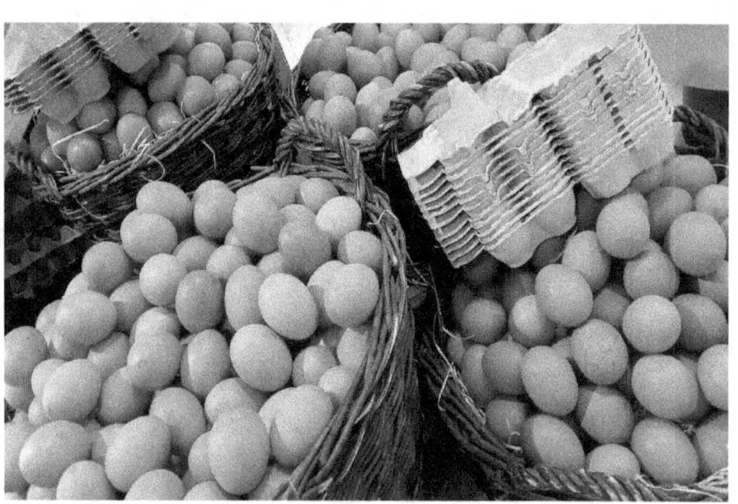

The History and Science Behind Carnivore Eating.

The history and science behind carnivore nutrition reflect the evolutionary roots of human dietary habits and the current scientific understanding of the nutritional consequences of consuming a diet primarily of animal foods. This section provides valuable insight into the reasons for adopting a carnivore diet and reveals its potential benefits and challenges.

As omnivores, humans have a long evolutionary history of consuming foods of plant and animal origin. Our early ancestors were hunters who gatherers diets depending on geography, climate, and available resources. It is widely accepted that animal foods have played an important role in human evolution, providing essential nutrients such as proteins, fats, vitamins, and minerals necessary for survival and optimal health.

Anthropological evidence suggests that our prehistoric ancestors relied heavily on animal foods, especially when plant foods were rare or less available. The ability to hunt and consume protein products may have contributed to the development of larger brains and the evolution of modern human physiology.

Nutritional Considerations

From a nutritional point of view, animal foods are a source of high-quality protein, essential fatty acids, vitamins (B12, A, D, K2, etc.), and minerals (iron, zinc, selenium, etc.). These nutrients are essential to support a variety of physiological functions, including muscle growth and repair, immune function, hormone synthesis, and cognitive health.

Pioneers of the carnivore diet argue that animal foods provide all essential nutrients in the most bioavailable form and are superior to plant foods in nutrient density and absorption. Evidence suggests that certain nutrients, such as vitamin B12 and heme iron, are more easily absorbed from animal than plant sources.

Although the carnivore diet remains controversial in the scientific community, several studies have investigated its potential health effects. Research in this area is limited, and results are often preliminary or based on anecdotal evidence rather than large clinical trials.

Some studies have shown that a carnivore diet may improve people's metabolic parameters, such as blood sugar, insulin sensitivity, and lipid profiles.

Anecdotal reports and case studies describe benefits such as weight loss, reduced inflammation, improved digestion, and increased mental clarity among adherents of the carnivore diet.

However, the long-term effects of carnivorous diets on health outcomes and disease risk remain uncertain, so it is important to interpret these results with caution.

Critics of the diet have expressed concern about the potential for nutritional deficiencies, particularly the essential micronutrients found in plant-based foods and the lack of fiber and phytonutrients that can contribute to overall health and well-being.

In conclusion, the history and science of carnivore nutrition provide exciting insights into the evolutionary and nutritional aspects of consuming a diet primarily of animal foods.

Although the carnivore diet may offer potential benefits, it raises issues and unanswered questions requiring further research and consideration. As with any dietary approach, evaluating the evidence, consulting a healthcare professional, and making an informed decision based on your health needs and preferences is essential.

Benefits and considerations

Exploring the carnivore diet's benefits and characteristics reveals its benefits and potential challenges, providing a nuanced understanding of this dietary approach and its impact on health and well-being.

Simplicity: The carnivore diet simplifies food choices by focusing primarily on animal foods, eliminating the need for complex meal planning and meal preparation associated with other diets.

Nutrient Density: Animal foods are rich in essential nutrients such as high-quality protein, vitamins, and minerals necessary for maintaining overall health, muscle growth, and metabolic function.

Potential for weight loss: Most people experience weight loss on a carnivore diet, which is associated with factors such as reduced caloric intake, increased satiety from high-protein foods, and improved metabolism.

Reduces inflammation: Eliminating plant foods that can cause inflammation from your diet may reduce inflammation and symptoms associated with autoimmune and digestive disorders in some people.

Improved Digestion: For people with digestive issues or sensitivities to certain plant foods, a carnivore diet can relieve symptoms by eliminating common triggers such as gluten, dairy, and high-fiber foods.

Increased mental clarity: Some proponents of the carnivore diet report improved cognitive function, concentration, and mental clarity and attribute these benefits to stabilizing blood sugar levels and reducing brain fog.

Our body and body system are different, so while most individuals may experience certain advantages of a carnivore's diet, others might not.

Nutritional adequacy: Carnivore diets may be lacking in certain nutrients found in plant-based foods, such as fiber, antioxidants, and phytonutrients, leading to potential nutritional deficiencies and long-term health effects. There are concerns about this.

Digestive problems: Transitioning to a carnivorous diet can be difficult for some people and can lead to digestive discomfort, constipation, and changes in intestinal function as the gut microbiome adapts to different food compositions.

Potential risks: Critics of the carnivore diet argue that the carnivore diet's potential risks include increased cholesterol levels, increased intake of saturated fat, and the long-term effects of eliminating entire food groups from the diet.

Social and practical considerations: A carnivorous diet differs significantly from usual dietary standards and may require special considerations, creating social problems and restrictions in social and restaurant settings.

Individual differences: Carnivore responses to diets vary significantly from individual to individual, and what works for one person may not necessarily work for another. It's essential to listen to your body and adjust your dietary approach based on your unique needs and preferences.

Lack of long-term study or research: Although anecdotal evidence and short-term studies indicate the potential benefits of the carnivore diet, there is a lack of long-term studies evaluating its safety, efficacy, and long-term sustainability.

Therefore, the carnivore diet includes potential benefits and considerations that should be carefully considered when considering this dietary approach.

While there may be some benefits, including simplicity, nutrient density, and potential for improvement in weight management and inflammation, there are also challenges related to nutritional adequacy, digestive health, and long-term sustainability.

CHAPTER TWO

Essential Tools and Equipment

Learning the basic tools and utensils needed for carnivorous meals is essential to ensure smooth meal preparation and cooking success. Whether you're a beginner or an experienced carnivore's dieter, having the right tools will simplify the cooking process and improve your overall cooking experience. The tools and equipment needed for a carnivore diet include:

High-Quality Knife: Buy a high-quality knife set, including a chef knife, boning knife, and paring knife. A sharp knife makes it easy to slice meat, cut steaks, and cook different cuts of beef precisely.

Cutting Board: Choose a durable wooden or plastic cutting board that provides a stable surface for cutting and slicing meat. Choose a large cutting board to accommodate different cuts of beef and minimize cross-contamination.

Meat thermometer: A meat thermometer is essential to ensure that your meat is cooked to the desired doneness and is safe to eat. Look for a digital meat thermometer with fast and accurate readings for the best results.

Cast Iron Skillet: Cast iron skillets are versatile kitchen tools perfect for searing steaks, cooking burgers, and roasting meats. Cast iron retains and conducts heat well, allowing you to sear your meat beautifully and with lots of flavor.

Grill or Grill Pan: If you love cooking outdoors, invest in a grill that perfectly grills steaks, burgers, and other meats. You can also use a grill pan indoors to add sear marks and a smoky flavor to meat dishes.

Dutch Oven: Dutch ovens are ideal for roasting large meats such as whole chickens, pot roasts, and pork shoulders. Choose a sturdy roasting pan with a rack to elevate the meat and allow air to circulate for even cooking.

Instant Pot or Slow Cooker: The Instant Pot or slow cooker prepares tender, flavorful meats with minimal effort. It makes hearty bone broths and stews and is perfect for carnivore-friendly meals.

Food processor or meat grinder: Food processors and meat grinders help grind meat, make homemade sausages, and make meat spreads and patties. Choose a durable, easy-to-clean model that meets your specific needs.

Meat tongs and fork: Tongs and meat forks are essential for moving and turning meat during cooking. Choose tongs with long handles and sturdy meat forks for added control and safety.

Storage Container: Purchase a variety of storage containers, including glass and plastic containers, resealable bags, and airtight containers, to store leftover meat, meal prep ingredients, and homemade sauces and condiments.

Equip your kitchen with these essential tools and equipment, and you'll be ready to embrace your carnivore diet with confidence and creativity. Whether you're grilling a steak, roasting a fish, roasting a whole chicken in the oven, or whipping up a hearty stew in the slow cooker, having the right tools at your disposal can enhance your culinary adventures.

Filling the kitchen

Equipping your kitchen for a carnivorous diet means stocking up on various high-quality animal products to suit your dietary needs and preferences. You can easily prepare delicious and nutritious meals by stocking your pantry, refrigerator, and freezer with carnivore-friendly ingredients. Here's a guide to stocking your kitchen with carnivores.

High-quality meat: Choose fresh, high-quality meat such as beef, pork, lamb, poultry (chicken, turkey), and fish. Choose grass-fed, pasture-raised, or organic foods whenever possible.

Seafood: Include fresh or frozen seafood in your diet, such as salmon, shrimp, tuna, cod, and shellfish. Look for wild-caught seafood from sustainable fisheries to ensure optimal quality and sustainability.

Eggs: Stock up on eggs, a versatile and nutrient-rich source of protein. Choose free-range or free-range eggs for better taste and nutritional value.

Bone Broth: Keep bone broth on hand for drinking, cooking, and flavoring soups, stews, and sauces. Consider making your bone broth or purchasing high-quality bone broth from a reputable brand.

Animal Fat: Animal fats such as beef tallow, lard, duck fat, and bacon fat are used to cook and flavor food. Process animal fat yourself or buy it in specialized stores or online stores.

Seasonings and Spices: Stock up on carnivore-friendly herbs and spices, such as salt, pepper, garlic powder, onion powder, dried herbs (rosemary, Thyme, oregano), and spices (paprika, cayenne pepper). Choose high-quality options without additives for optimal taste.

Seasonings: Look for seasonings without sugar or additives, such as mustard, hot sauce, mayonnaise, or vinegar, to enhance the flavor of your dishes. Check ingredient labels carefully to avoid hidden sugars and additives.

Refrigerator basics

Fresh Meats: Store fresh meats such as steaks, roasts, ground beef, and chicken in the refrigerator for easy access when preparing meals. To avoid cross-contamination, store meat tightly closed and on lower shelves.

Dairy products (optional): If you want, include dairy products such as butter, cheese, and heavy cream in your carnivore's diet. Choose high-quality, full-fat dairy products made from grass-fed or grass-fed animals.

Eggs: To maintain freshness and quality, keep eggs in the refrigerator. Eggs should be stored in their original packaging to avoid absorbing odors and flavors from other foods.

Bone broth: Homemade or store-bought bone broth can be stored in the refrigerator for up to a week or frozen longer. Thaw frozen bone broth in the fridge before using it in a recipe.

Freezer basics

Frozen meat: Store a variety of frozen meats such as steaks, roasts, ground meat, and seafood in the freezer for long-term storage. Pack meat in airtight containers or freezer bags to prevent freezer burn.

Frozen seafood: Store frozen seafood such as shrimp, fish fillets, and shellfish in the freezer for easy access when needed. Thaw frozen seafood in the refrigerator or under running water before cooking.

Prepared meals (optional): Consider preparing and freezing carnivore-friendly meals like meatballs, burgers, stews, and soups for quick and convenient convenience. Prepared meals can be individually packaged for easy reheating and portion control.

With these carnivore-friendly essentials in your kitchen, you'll have everything you need to prepare delicious and satisfying meals that support the carnivore lifestyle. With a fully equipped kitchen, you can experience simple and rich carnivorous cooking while enjoying the many benefits that carnivorous cooking has to offer.

Shopping Tips for Carnivores

Buying carnivorous products means avoiding plant products and focusing primarily on animal products. Here are some shopping tips to help you find quality meat, seafood, and other essential ingredients for your carnivore's diet.

Choose high-quality meat: Look for grass-fed beef, pasture-raised chicken, and wild-caught seafood whenever possible. These options generally offer superior taste, nutritional content, and ethical sourcing compared to conventionally raised meat.

Choose fresh, whole meat: Whenever possible, choose fresh meat from the butcher counter or meat aisle rather than pre-packaged meat. Whole cuts, such as steaks, roasts, and whole chickens, are more flexible in meal preparation and are of higher quality.

Check the label carefully: When purchasing packaged meat and seafood, read the labels carefully to ensure they contain minimal additives and preservatives. Avoid foods with added sugar, fillers, artificial flavors, and other unnecessary ingredients.

Buy in bulk: Consider buying meat in bulk, especially if you can access a freezer for long-term storage. Buying more often means you save money and ensure you always have carnivore-friendly food. Take a look at specialty stores and butcher shops.

Visit specialty butchers, farmers markets, and local farms to find a wide variety of high-quality meats, including specialty cuts, organ meats, and grass-fed products.

Developing relationships with local producers can also provide access to premium meats and personalized service.

Stock up on pantry staples: Keep carnivore staples like eggs, bacon, butter, and bone broth in your pantry and refrigerator for convenient, ready-to-eat snacks. These versatile ingredients can be used in various recipes and provide valuable nutrients for a complete carnivore diet.

Consider online options: Check out online retailers and subscription services specializing in grass-fed meat, sustainable seafood, and other carnivore-friendly products. Ordering online makes it easy to select and obtain specialty items that may not be available locally.

Keep your budget in mind: High-quality meat and seafood can be expensive, but there are ways carnivores can buy them more economically. Consider looking for sales, discounts, and bulk buying options to choose the most nutritious cuts of meat within your budget. Plan your meals.

Before you go to the supermarket, plan your meals for the week to ensure you stock up on the ingredients you need and avoid food waste.

Meal planning can also help you stay focused on your dietary goals and resist the temptation to deviate from a carnivorous lifestyle.

Change your shopping habits: Switching to a carnivorous diet may require changing your shopping habits and mindset. Focus on filling your shopping cart with nutritious animal foods while minimizing or eliminating purchases of processed and plant-based foods.

By following these shopping tips for carnivores, you'll be ready to confidently roam your grocery store or market and find the highest quality meat, seafood, and other essential ingredients that support your carnivore lifestyle.

Chapter 3

Meat preparation and selection

Choose High-Quality Meats

High-quality meat is essential to providing your carnivores journey with delicious, nutritious, and satisfying meals. Here are some tips for choosing the best meat for your carnivorous lifestyle.

Grass-fed beef or Pasture raised: Choose grass-fed beef and grass-fed meat whenever possible. These animals are typically raised in a more natural environment, have access to Pasture, and may have a higher nutritional profile than traditionally raised animals.

Look for marbling: Marbling refers to the intramuscular fat distributed throughout the meat, giving it flavor and tenderness. Choose cuts with visible marbling to make your food juicier and more flavorful.

Check color and texture: Fresh meat should be bright in color and firm in texture. Avoid meat that is discolored, slippery, or has an unpleasant odor, as this may indicate spoilage or poor quality.

Consider aging: Some cuts of meat, such as beef, are better when aged, as they become more tender and flavorful. For the best quality, look for appropriately aged meat (by dry aging or wet aging).

Check the label: Read the label carefully to understand how the animal was raised and what it was fed. Look for terms like "grass-fed," "pasture-fed," "organic," and "hormone-free" to help you choose high-quality meat.

Choose whole meat: Whenever possible, choose whole meat over processed or packaged meat. Whole cuts tend to be fresher and less processed because you have more control over how they are cooked.

Consider organ meats: Don't underestimate the nutritional value of organ meats, which are packed with essential vitamins, minerals, and nutrients. Include organ meats like liver, heart, and kidneys in your diet for variety and nutritional diversity.

Ask your butcher: Build a relationship with your local butcher or meat supplier, and feel free to ask questions about meat sourcing, quality, and recommendations for different cuts. Your butcher will provide valuable information and recommendations to help you choose the best meat.

Keep your budget in mind: High-quality meat can be expensive, but there are ways to make informed choices that stay within your budget. Consider choosing the cuts that offer the best value for money regarding taste, nutritional value, and versatility.

Consider sustainable options: Choose meat from sources that prioritize sustainability and ethical animal welfare principles where possible. Supporting responsible and environmentally conscious producers helps promote a more sustainable food system.

Basic Cooking Methods

Mastering basic cooking techniques is essential to creating flavorful meat dishes on a carnivore diet. Here are some basic cooking techniques to help you improve your cooking skills.

Searing involves cooking meat over high heat to create a flavorful outer skin while retaining moisture. Heat a skillet or grill to sear the meat, then add the beef and sear for a few minutes until browned on all sides.

Grilled: Grilling is a popular cooking method that imparts a smoky flavor to meat while leaving attractive sear marks. Preheat the grill to medium heat, season the meat, and cook directly over the heat or coals until the desired doneness is achieved.

Roasting involves cooking meat in the oven at high temperatures to create a tender and flavorful dish. To roast the beef, preheat the oven, season the meat with herbs and spices, and place on a rack in a casserole dish. Cook until the internal temperature reaches the desired doneness.

Fry in a frying pan: Pan-frying is a versatile cooking method that involves cooking meat in a pot of oil or fat. To brown the beef, heat the oil or shortening in a skillet over medium heat, add the meat, and fry until browned and cooked through, turning as needed.

Roasting: Roasting is cooking meat by exposing it to high heat from above. To sear the beef, preheat the Dutch oven, season it, and place it on a baking sheet or rack. Grill the meat under the grill until browned and to your desired doneness. Cook slowly. Slow cooking is great for tenderizing tough cuts of meat and adding flavor. To slow-cook meat, place it in a slow cooker or Dutch oven with liquid and seasonings and cook over low heat for several hours until the meat is tender and falls apart quickly. Sous vide: Sous vide is a cooking method that involves cooking meat in a water bath at a specific temperature for an extended period. To sous vide meat, vacuum seal the meat in a seasoning bag and cook in a sous vide machine or immersion oven until cooked.

Grill: Grilling involves cooking meat on a flat, heated surface like a skillet or griddle. To grill meat, heat a skillet or griddle, season the meat, and cook until browned and cooked through, turning as needed. Braising: Braising is a cooking method in which meat is fried in oil and then slowly cooked in liquid until tender. To stew the meat, sear it in a pan and transfer it to the pan along with the liquid and flavorings. Cover and simmer over low heat until the meat is tender.

Smoking: Smoking is a cooking method that gives the meat a rich, smoky flavor. To smoke meat, preheat your smoker or grill it with wood chips, season it, and place it in the smoker. Simmer until the meat is tender and develops a smoky flavor. Once you master these fundamental cooking techniques, even carnivores will be ready to prepare various delicious and flavorful meat dishes. Whether you're grilling steaks, burgers, or slow-cooking stir-fries, these techniques will yield mouth-watering results every time.

Improved flavor and seasoning

Although carnivore diets are primarily focused on animal foods, there are still many ways to enhance the flavor of food using seasonings and other flavorings. Here are some carnivore-friendly flavorings and seasonings to consider.

Salt is an essential seasoning that brings out meat's natural flavor and adds depth to dishes. Choose high-quality sea salt or Himalayan salt to season your meat.

Pepper: Ground black pepper adds spiciness and complexity to meat dishes. For optimal taste and aroma, use freshly ground pepper.

Garlic powder: Garlic powder is an all-purpose seasoning that adds flavor to meat dishes without using raw garlic. Sprinkle liberally on steaks, roasts, and burgers to add depth of flavor.

Onion powder: Onion powder adds a subtle sweetness and flavor to meat dishes and is a popular seasoning among carnivores. Use to season ground meat, meatballs, and marinades.

Paprika: Paprika adds color and a sweet, smoky flavor to meat dishes. Smoked paprika adds depth and complexity to dishes.

Cayenne pepper: For those who like spicy food, cayenne pepper adds a spicy kick to meat dishes. Use sparingly to add spiciness so as not to overpower other flavors.

Dried herbs: Dried herbs such as rosemary, Thyme, and oregano can be used to season and add flavor to meat. Experiment with different herb combinations to find your favorite flavor profile.

Steak Seasoning: Commercial steak seasonings often contain blends of salt, pepper, garlic, and other herbs and spices designed to enhance the flavor of steak and other meats. Look for a steak seasoning blend that doesn't contain sugar or artificial ingredients.

Butter: Butter adds richness and flavor to meat dishes, mainly as a spread or finishing touch. Choose high-quality grass-fed butter for the best flavor and nutritional value.

Fresh herbs (optional): Carnivore diets primarily focus on animal foods, but some people add small amounts of fresh herbs, such as parsley, coriander, and green onions, to add color and freshness to their meals. When using seasonings and flavor enhancers in your carnivore's diet, choosing products without added sugars, fillers, or artificial ingredients is essential. Experiment with combinations and techniques to discover new flavor profiles and get the most out of your carnivore-friendly dishes.

Chapter 4

Breakfast

Simple Steak and Eggs

Ingredient:

- One boneless steak (ribeye, sirloin, New York strip, etc.)
- 2-3 eggs
- Pepper
- Salt
- Butter or Ghee
- Optional: fresh herbs for garnish (such as parsley or chives).

Instructions:

Prepare the steak:

- Remove the steak from the refrigerator and let it come to room temperature for about 30 minutes.

- Pat steak with paper towels to remove excess moisture. Carefully sprinkle both sides of the steak with salt and pepper.

Cook the steak:

- Preheat a cast iron skillet or grill over high heat. Make sure your skillet or grill is hot enough before adding the steak.

- Add one tablespoon of butter or ghee to the skillet or grill. Carefully place the seasoned steak on a hot surface.

- Grill the steak for 3-4 minutes on each side for medium-rare doneness, or adjust the cooking time to suit your preference. Check the internal temperature of the steak using a meat thermometer. For medium-rare cooking, the internal temperature should be approximately 130-135°F (55-57°C). Once the steak is done to your liking, please remove it from the pan or grill and let it sit on the cutting board for a few minutes.

Cook the eggs:

- While the steak is cooling, cook the eggs. Cooking the eggs in the same skillet you used to sear the steak allows them to absorb the delicious juices.

- Crack the eggs into the skillet, golden side up, and cook lightly or scrambled, depending on your preference.

- Add a pinch of salt and pepper to the eggs.

Serve:

- Cut the rested steak against the grain into thin slices.

- Place steak slices and eggs on a plate.

- Garnish with fresh herbs, if desired. Serve immediately and enjoy an easy and satisfying steak and eggs.

This classic carnivore-friendly dish is perfect for breakfast, brunch, or any day you crave a hearty, flavorful protein meal. Adjust seasoning amounts and the time for cooking to your taste, and feel free to add your favorite herbs and spices to your dish.

Bacon Sausage

Ingredients:

- Eight sausages of your choice (pork, beef, chicken, etc.)
- Toothpick or skewer
- Eight pieces bacon
- Olive oil (optional for grease)

Instructions:

Preheat oven:

- Preheat oven to 400°F (200°C). Line a baking sheet with parchment paper or foil for easier cleanup.

Wrap the sausage:

- Takes each sausage one at a time and wraps them tightly around the bacon slices, overlapping them slightly to secure them in place.
- Secure the ends of the bacon with toothpicks or skewers to prevent it from fraying while cooking.
- Optional: Brush with olive oil (optional): If you prefer, brush the bacon-wrapped sausages with olive oil and brown them in the oven.

Cooking bacon sausage:

- Place the bacon-wrapped sausages evenly apart on the prepared baking sheet to ensure they cook evenly.

- Transfer the skillet to the preheated oven and bake for 20 to 25 minutes, or until the bacon is crispy and the sausage is cooked.

- Flip the sausages halfway through cooking to ensure even cooking on all sides.

- Serve: Once cooked, remove the bacon-wrapped sausages from the oven and let them cool slightly.

- Carefully remove toothpicks or skewers before eating.

- Serve bacon-wrapped sausages with your favorite sauces and seasonings as a delicious appetizer, appetizer, or main dish.

These bacon-wrapped sausages make a popular appetizer or main dish, perfect for get-togethers, game days, or any time you want a delicious and filling snack. Feel free to customize the recipe using your favorite type of sausage and experiment with different seasonings and sauces for added flavor. Enjoy the perfect combination of crispy bacon and juicy sausage in every bite.

Sizzling Breakfast Skillet

Ingredients

- Four pieces of bacon (chopped)
- Four eggs, preferably large
- One medium onion (chopped)
- 1 pound breakfast sausage (crushed)
- One bell pepper (any color), chopped
- Two cloves of garlic (minced)
- salt and pepper for taste
- Optional: Fresh herbs for garnish (such as parsley or chives).

How to cook:

- Prepare the bacon: Heat a large cast iron skillet over medium heat. Add the chopped bacon to the skillet and cook, stirring occasionally, until crispy. Once cooked, remove the bacon from the pan, leaving the melted fat in the pan.

- **Prepare the sausage:** Add crumbled breakfast sausage to the same pot with bacon grease. Cook the sausage over medium heat, breaking it up with a spatula, until browned and cooked.

- **Add vegetables**: When the sausage is ready, add the chopped onions and peppers to the pan. Cook for 3 to 4 minutes or until vegetables are soft and begin to caramelize.

- **Add garlic**: Add the minced garlic and cook for another 1-2 minutes or until it starts bringing out an aroma.

- **Create a hole in the sausage for the egg:** Use a spatula to make four indentations in the sausage and vegetable mixture. Crack an egg into each well, careful not to break the yolk.

- **Prepare the eggs:** Cover the skillet and cook the eggs over medium-low heat for 5 to 7 minutes, or until the whites are set and the yolks are consistent the way you like. If you prefer a firmer yolk, cook for a few more minutes.

- **Finish cooking the food and serve:** Sprinkle the cooked bacon bits onto the skillet once the eggs are cooked to your liking. Season the entire pot with salt and pepper. Garnish with fresh herbs, if desired. Serve hot breakfast bread straight from the pan so everyone has their share. Enjoy the delicious combination of flavorful sausage, crispy bacon, and perfectly cooked eggs.

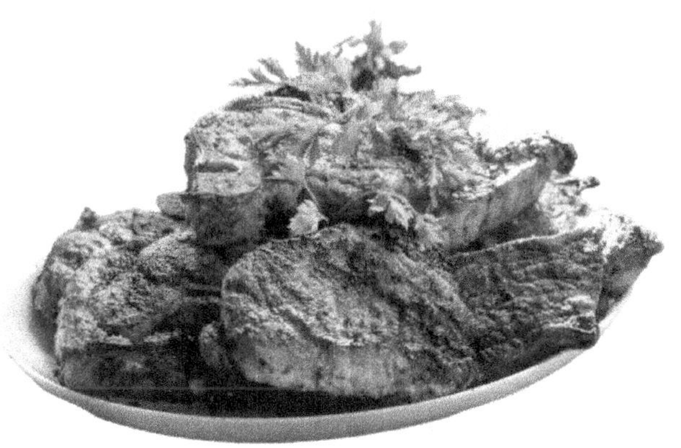

This piping hot Carnivore Breakfast Skillet is a delicious and satisfying option for those on a carnivore diet. Packed with protein and nutrients, it's a delightful way to start your day and fill your body with healthy ingredients. Feel free to customize your recipes with carnivore-friendly ingredients and enjoy a satisfying breakfast that will keep you full until lunch.

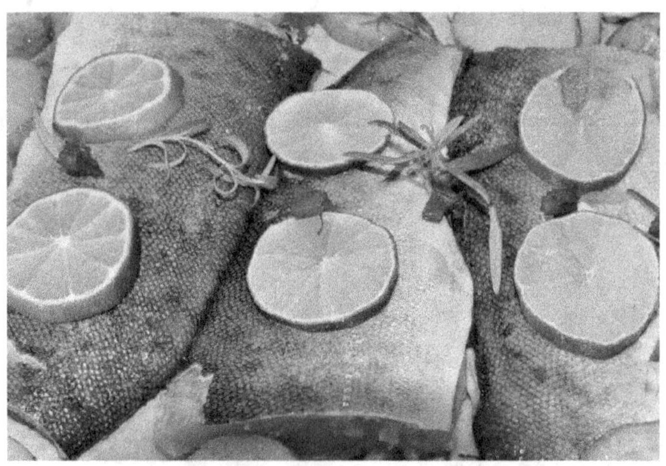

Chapter 5

Lunch

Classic Beef Burger

Ingredients:

- 1 pound ground beef (preferably 80/20 blended)
- Four hamburger buns or burger bum
- Salt and Pepper Taste
- You can add any stuffing of your choice, for example, Sliced cheese (cheddar, American, Swiss, etc.).
- Lettuce leaves
- Sliced tomato
- Chopped onion
- Pickles
- Ketchup, mustard, mayonnaise, or your favorite toppings.

How to cook:

- **Prepare the grill (or pan):** Preheat the grill to medium-high heat. If using a frying pan, heat it on the stove over medium-high heat.

- **Form the chop**: Divide the ground beef into four equal parts and shape each into a round patty about 3/4 to 1 inch thick. Use your thumb to make a slight indentation in the center of each patty. This will prevent the hamburger from expanding during cooking.

Season the Patties:

- Season both sides of each patty carefully with salt and pepper or your favorite seasoning blend. Prepare the cutlets.

- **Cook the patties:** Place seasoned hamburger patties on a preheated grill or skillet. Bake for about 4 to 5 minutes, without touching the top, until the top is nicely browned. Flip the cutlets with a spatula and continue cooking for 3 to 4 minutes or until the internal temperature reaches the desired level of doneness.

- For medium-rare cooking: 130-135°F (55-57°C).
- For Medium: 140-145°F (60-63°C)
- Moderate to Good: 150-155°F (65-68°C)
- For best cooking: 160°F (71°C) or higher.

If you're adding cheese, place a slice on top of each patty during the last few minutes of cooking, then cover the grill or pan and wait until the cheese melts.

- **Toasting the buns:** While the patties cook, lightly toast the hamburger buns on the grill or in a skillet until golden brown. Assemble the burgers. Place the cooked hamburger patty on the bottom of the toasted bun. Add your favorite toppings like lettuce, tomatoes, onions, pickles, and seasonings. Finally, place the top bun on top of each burger.

- **Serve and enjoy:** Serve the classic beef burger hot immediately for a juicy, flavorful meal.

Customize the classic beef burger with your favorite toppings and seasonings to suit your preferences. Whether starting a barbecue grill in the backyard or cooking for yourself on the stove, these homemade burgers or hamburgers are the best to share with your family and friends.

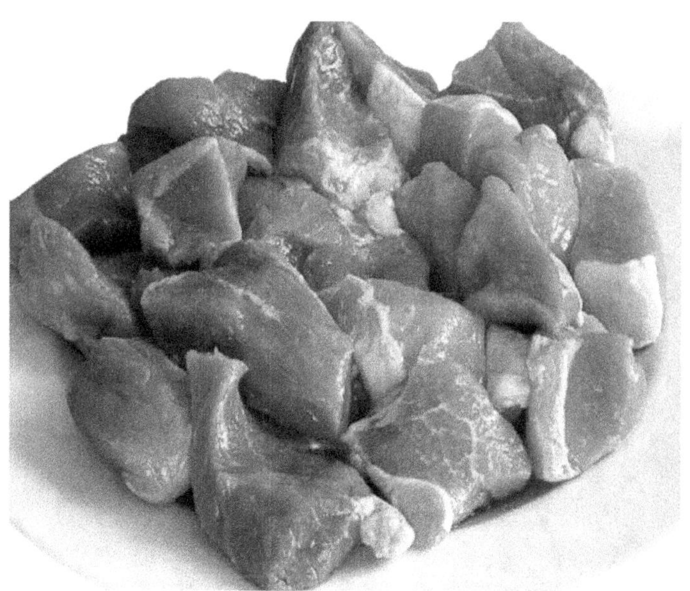

Grilled Chicken Ceasar Salad

Ingredients to use: In the case of fried chicken:

- 2 Chicken breasts without skin and boneless
- Two tablespoons of olive oil
- Salt and pepper for Taste
- One teaspoon of garlic powder
- One teaspoon of dry oregano
- One teaspoon of Thyme (dried)
- Juice 1 lemon

Ingredient to make the Ceasar Dressing:

1/2 mayonnaise cup

Two tablespoons of parmesan with grated cheese

Two teaspoons of Dijon mustard

Garlic clove 2, chopped

Two tablespoons of freshly compressed lemon juice

1 cup of water shire sauce

Salt and pepper for taste

- **For salad:**

One large romaine lettuce head, chopped

1/4 cup of grated cheese and parmesan

Food group (optional)

Instruction on how to make:

Tips on how to prepare the chicken:

- Season the chicken breasts with salt, pepper, garlic, dried oregano, and dried Thyme.

- Drizzle the seasoned chicken breasts with olive oil and lemon juice, and make sure they are evenly coated.

- Preheat the grill to medium-high heat. Grill the chicken breasts for 6 to 8 minutes per side or until cooked through and no longer pink in the center.

- Remove from the grill and let rest for a few minutes before slicing.

How to Prepare Caesar Dressing:

- Whisk the mayonnaise in a small bowl, grate Parmesan, Dijon mustard, minced garlic, lemon juice, Worcestershire sauce, salt, and pepper until smooth.

- Please adjust the seasoning to your preference.

Arranging the salad:

- Toss chopped romaine lettuce with Caesar dressing in a large bowl until evenly coated.

- Transfer the dressed salad to a plate or bowl.

- Slice the grilled chicken breast and place on top of the salad for garnish.

- Sprinkle the salad with grated Parmesan cheese.

- If desired, top with croutons for added texture and crunch.

Serve:

- Serve the Grilled Chicken Caesar Salad immediately and have everyone mix the ingredients before enjoying.
- Garnish with additional lemon wedges to garnish the salad, if desired.

Grilled Chicken Caesar Salad is a flavorful and satisfying dish perfect for lunch or dinner. The combination of tender grilled chicken, crunchy romaine lettuce, and creamy Caesar dressing creates a classic flavor that will delight your Taste buds. Enjoy this salad, or pair it with your favorite breads and side dishes for a complete meal.

Tuna and Avocado Boat

Ingredients to use:

- Two ripe avocados
- One can (5 oz) tuna, drained
- 2-3 tablespoons mayonnaise (check for sugar-free options)
- Salt and pepper for taste
- Optional: Add lemon juice for added flavor.

Instructions on how to make:

Preparing the avocado:

- Cut the avocado in half lengthwise and remove the seed. S
- coop the pulp from the avocado halves to create a large cavity and boat shape.
- Save the collected pulp for another use or throw it away.

Preparing the tuna stuffing:

- Add drained tuna and mayonnaise to a bowl and mix.

- Mix well until the mayonnaise is evenly coated on the tuna.

- Add salt and pepper to the tuna mixture for taste.

- Adjust seasoning as needed.

- You can also add a little lemon juice for extra flavor if you like.

Fill the hole made on avocado:

- Pour the tuna mixture into the cavity of each avocado half, distributing it evenly between them

- . Press gently to fill the boat with avocado completely.

Serve:

- Serve Tuna and Avocado Boats immediately to enjoy a hearty, carnivore-friendly meal.

- Enjoy creamy tuna and rich buttery avocado for a nutritious and flavorful snack or light meal.

- These tuna and avocado boats are perfect for beginners following a carnivore diet and are a delicious and convenient way to incorporate nutrient-dense ingredients into your diet.

- This dish requires minimal prep and cleanup, making it an excellent option for those looking for a quick and easy meal for their carnivore.

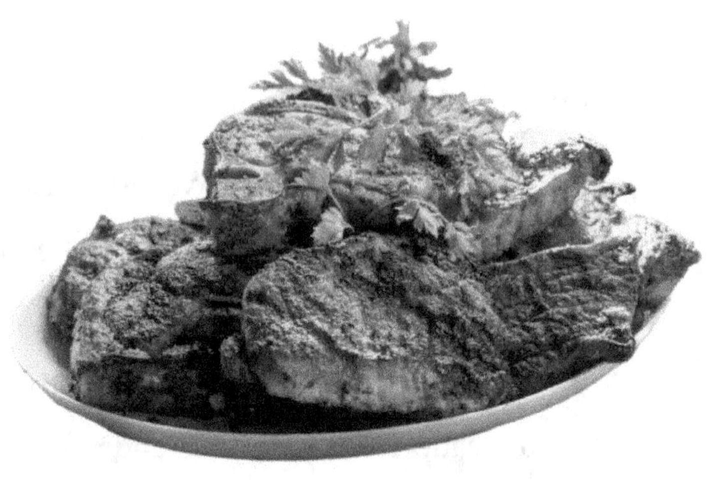

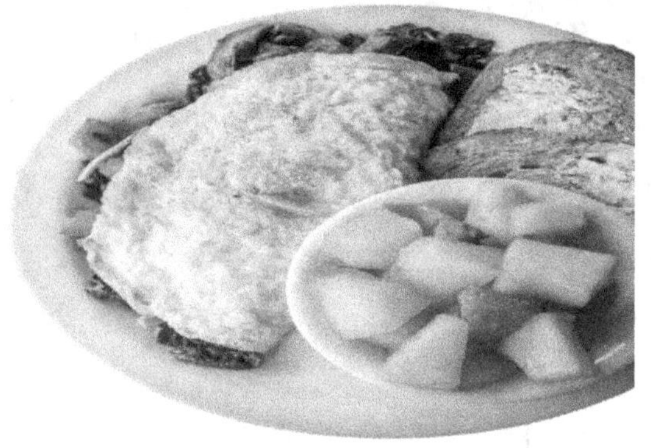

Chapter 6

Dinner

Ribeye Steak with Garlic butter

Ingredients to use:

- Two ribeye steaks, about 1 inch thick
- salt and pepper Taste
- Two tablespoons unsalted butter
- Two cloves of garlic (minced)
- Optional: fresh herbs for garnish (such as Thyme or rosemary).

Instructions on how to make:

How to Prepare the Steak:

- Remove the ribeye from the refrigerator and let it cool to room temperature for about 30 minutes. This ensures more even cooking.

- Pat steak with paper towels to remove excess moisture.

- Season each steak carefully with salt and pepper on both sides.

Cooking of the steak:

- Preheat a cast iron skillet or grill over high heat.

- Make sure your skillet or grill is hot enough before adding the steak.

- Place the seasoned ribeye steak on a hot griddle or grill. For medium-rare, cook for 3 to 4 minutes on each side, or adjust the cooking time according to your desired doneness.

- Check the internal temperature of the steak using a meat thermometer. For medium-rare cooking, the internal temperature should be approximately 130-135°F (55-57°C).

- Once the steak is done to your liking, please remove it from the pan or grill and let it cool on a cutting board for a few minutes.

Preparing the garlic butter:

- While the steak is cooling, melt the unsalted butter in a small skillet over medium heat.

- Add the minced garlic to the melted butter and cook for 1 to 2 minutes or until the garlic is fragrant and lightly browned.

- Be careful not to burn the garlic. Remove the pot from the heat and set aside.

Serving:

- Transfer the rested ribeye to a plate. Pour the garlic butter over each steak and let it melt to coat the surface.

- Garnish with fresh herbs such as Thyme or rosemary for added flavor and presentation if desired.

- Serving the ribeye steak immediately while it's still hot is the best, garnished with garlic butter.

Enjoy a juicy, flavorful ribeye steak coated in garlic butter and perfectly seasoned. This Garlic Butter Ribeye Steak recipe is simple but delicious, making it perfect for those new to the carnivore diet.

With just a few ingredients and minimal preparation, you can enjoy a delicious steak dinner that will satisfy your carnivorous cravings.

Pork chops braised with herbs

Ingredients to make use of:

- Four bone-in pork chops, about 1 inch thick
- salt and pepper Taste
- Two tablespoons of olive oil
- Two cloves of garlic (minced)
- One teaspoon of dried Thyme
- One teaspoon of dried rosemary
- One teaspoon dried oregano
- Optional: Fresh herbs for garnish (such as parsley or Thyme).

Instructions on how to make:

Preheating in oven: Preheat oven to 400°F (200°C).

Preparing the pork chops: Pat pork chops dry with paper towels to remove excess moisture. Carefully sprinkle both sides of the pork chops with salt and pepper.

Preparing the herb mixture:

- Add olive oil, minced garlic, dried Thyme, rosemary, and oregano to make an herb mixture in a small bowl.

Cover with pork chops:

- Brush both sides of each pork chop with the herb mixture and coat it evenly.

Cook and roast the pork chops:

- Place seasoned pork chops on a baking sheet lined with parchment or foil paper.

- Transfer the baking sheet to the preheated oven and bake the pork chops for about 20 to 25 minutes, or until the internal temperature reaches 145°F (63°C).

- Cooking time may vary depending on the thickness of the pork chops, so use a meat thermometer to check for doneness.

Cooling and Serving of the food: Once cooked, remove the pork chops from the oven and let them rest for a few minutes before serving.

Garnish with fresh herbs such as parsley or Thyme for flavor and presentation if desired.

Serve our herb-roasted pork chops hot and enjoy the tender, flavorful meat. These herb-roasted pork chops are easy to prepare yet full of flavor, perfect for beginners on a carnivorous diet. These pork chops will complement any meal with a delicious blend of herbs and spices. Pair with your favorite low-carb side dishes for a hearty and healthy lunch.

Fried salmon fillet

Ingredient to make use of:

- Four skinless salmon fillets, about 6 ounces each
- salt and pepper Taste
- Two tablespoons olive oil or ghee
- Optional: lemon wedges for Serving.

Instructions on how to make:

How to Prepare the Salmon:

- Dry the salmon fillets with paper towels to remove excess moisture.
- This creates a crispy dough.

Seasoning of the salmon:

- Season both sides of the salmon fillet carefully with salt and pepper.

Preheating the pot:

- Heat a large skillet over medium-high heat.
- Add olive oil or ghee and stir to coat the bottom of the pan evenly.

Frying the Salmon:

- Once the pot is hot, carefully place the salmon fillets, skin side down, in the pot.

- Please be careful, as oil may splatter.

Cooking the Salmon Fillets:

- Cook the salmon fillets, without stirring, for about 4 to 5 minutes or until the skin is crisp and golden brown.

- This will help the skin adhere to the pan and prevent it from sticking.

- Carefully flip the salmon fillets using a spatula and cook for another 3 to 4 minutes until the flesh is opaque and flakes easily with a fork.

- The internal temperature must reach 145°F (63°C) to cook salmon.

Serving:

- Transfer the seared salmon fillets to a plate. If desired, squeeze fresh lemon juice over the salmon fillets for brightness and flavor.

- Enjoy the fried salmon piping hot.

This pan-fried salmon fillet recipe is quick and easy and perfect for those new to the carnivore diet. With minimal ingredients and preparation, you can enjoy delicious, nutritious salmon fillets that are crispy on the outside and soft on the inside. Serve with your favorite low-carb vegetables or enjoy on its own for a hearty lunch.

Chapter 7

Side Dishes

Creamy Cauliflower Puree

Materials and Ingredients to use:

- One cauliflower (large head), cut into florets
- Two tablespoons unsalted butter or ghee
- Two cloves of garlic (minced)
- 1/4 cup fresh cream
- Salt and pepper for taste
- Optional: minced garlic or parsley for garnish.

Instructions on how to make:

Steamed cauliflower:

- Place the cauliflower florets in a steaming basket set over a pot of boiling water. Cover and steam for 10-12 minutes or until cauliflower is tender when pierced with a fork.

Drain and dry the cauliflower:

- Once the cauliflower is cooked, please remove it from the steamer and drain excess water. Place the cauliflower on a clean kitchen towel or paper towel to absorb any remaining moisture.

Blending of the cauliflower:

- Transfer the steamed cauliflower to a food processor or blender.

- Add unsalted butter or ghee, minced garlic, and heavy cream to the cauliflower.

- Blend until smooth and creamy, scraping down the sides of the processor or blender as needed. If the mixture is too thick, you may need to add a little cream.

- Season the creamy cauliflower puree with salt and pepper. Adjust seasoning as needed.

Serving of Creamy Cauliflower Puree

- Transfer the creamy cauliflower puree to a bowl.

- Garnish with chopped onion or parsley for added flavor and presentation if desired.

- Serve the creamy cauliflower puree warm for a delicious and nutritious side dish.

This creamy cauliflower mash is a delicious, low-carb alternative to traditional mashed potatoes, perfect for those on a carnivorous diet. With its velvety texture and rich flavor, it goes well with various meat dishes, making it a satisfying addition to any dish. Enjoy this creamy cauliflower puree as a comforting, healthy addition to your carnivore menu.

Bacon and brussels sprouts

Ingredients to use:

- 1 pound Brussels sprouts (trimmed and cut in half)
- Four pieces of bacon (chopped)
- Two tablespoons unsalted butter or ghee
- salt and pepper Taste
- Optional: grated Parmesan cheese to garnish.

Instructions on how to make:

Preparing the bacon:

- In a large skillet, fry the chopped bacon over medium heat until crispy.
- Remove the crispy bacon from the pan, leaving the bacon fat in the pan.

Preparing the Brussels sprouts:

- Add the halved Brussels sprouts to the same pot as the bacon fat.

- Cook Brussels sprouts over medium heat, stirring occasionally, until browned and lightly caramelized, about 8 to 10 minutes.

Mixing with bacon:

- Return the bacon to the pot once the Brussels sprouts are cooked to your liking.

- Stir to infuse the bacon flavor into the Brussels sprouts.

Adding butter:

- Add unsalted or melted butter to the pot with the Brussels sprouts and bacon.
- Stir until butter melts and Brussels sprouts are evenly coated.

Seasoning and Serving of the Bacon and Brussels sprouts:

- Season bacon and Brussels sprouts with salt and pepper.

- Be careful with the amount of salt, as the bacon may be salty.

- Garnish with grated Parmesan cheese for added flavor, if desired.

- Transfer the Brussels sprouts and bacon to a platter and serve warm for a flavorful side dish.

This bacon Brussels sprouts recipe is a delicious and satisfying option for those on a carnivorous diet. The combination of the rich flavor of bacon and caramelized Brussels sprouts allows you to enjoy vegetables while maintaining your meat-eating habits. Serve these bacon Brussels sprouts with your favorite meat for a hearty and healthy lunch.

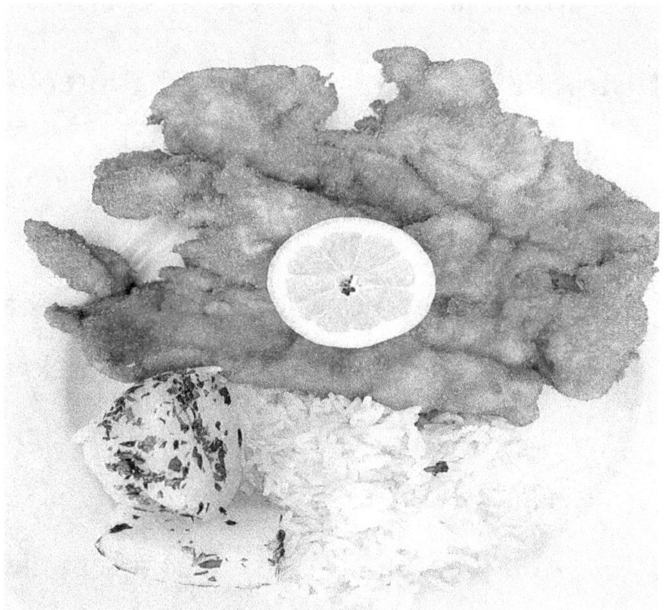

Buttered Asparagus Spears:

Ingredients to make use of:

- 1 pound asparagus spears, tough ends cut off
- Two tablespoons unsalted butter or ghee
- Salt and pepper for taste
- Optional: lemon wedges for Serving.

Instructions on making Buttered Asparagus Spears:

- Steam the asparagus.
- Fill a large pot with a few inches of water and place the steamer basket inside. Bring water to a boil over high heat.
- Add the trimmed asparagus tips to the steamer basket. Cover and steam for

about 4-5 minutes or until the asparagus is tender but crispy.

Shock the asparagus:

- Once the asparagus is cooked, transfer it to a bowl of ice water to stop it from cooking.
- This will maintain the bright green color and crunchy texture of the asparagus.

Drain and dry the asparagus:

- Remove the asparagus from the ice water and drain well.
- Dry the spears with paper towels to remove excess moisture.

Roasting the asparagus:

- Melt the unsalted butter or ghee in a large skillet over medium heat.

- Add the steamed asparagus spears to the pot and arrange in a single layer.

- Cook asparagus, stirring occasionally, until heated through and lightly coated with butter, 2 to 3 minutes.

- Season the buttered asparagus spears with salt and pepper. Adjust seasoning as needed.

Serving the Bacon and Brussels sprouts:

- Transfer the buttered asparagus spears to a plate.

- Garnish with lemon wedges if desired to add more flavor to the asparagus.

- Serve the buttered asparagus spears warm for a flavorful and nutritious side dish.

These buttered asparagus spears make a simple, elegant side dish that pairs perfectly with various meat dishes. With its crispy texture and delicate taste, it is sure to be a great addition to any meal. Enjoy a healthy and satisfying lunch with carnivore favorites.

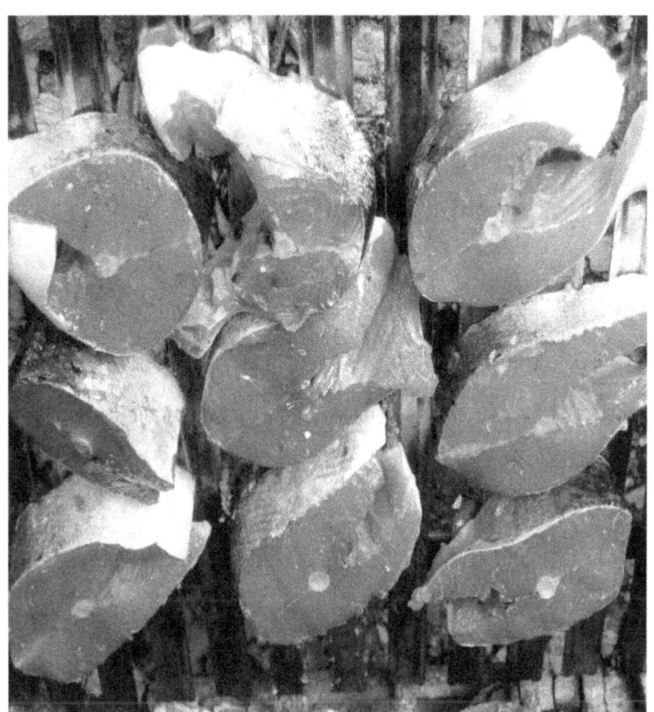

Chapter 8

Appetizers and Snacks

Beef Jerky

Ingredient to use:

- One pound of beef (flank or round steak) is thinly sliced against the grain.

- 1/4 cup soy sauce (or coconut amino for options that do not contain gluten)

- Worcestershire sauce two tablespoons

- Apple cider one tablespoon

- One teaspoon of garlic powder

- One teaspoon of onion powder

- One teaspoon of black Pepper

- 1/2 teaspoon of smoked paprika (optional, additional taste)

- If you like, you can add a pinch of red pepper flakes to heat

How to make:

How to marinade:

- In the bowl, mix soy sauce, Worcestershire sauce, apple cider vinegar, garlic powder, onion, black pepper, smoked paprika (if used), and red pepper flakes (as needed). Mix well and combine.

Marinate the beef:

- Place the thinly sliced beef in a resealable plastic bag or shallow dish.
- Pour the marinade over the beef, ensuring all slices are evenly coated.
- Rub the marinade over the beef to maximize flavor penetration.

- Seal the bag or cover the mold with plastic wrap and refrigerate until flavor develops, at least 4 hours, preferably overnight.

Preheat in your oven or dehydrator:

- Preheat to the lowest temperature possible (usually around 150-170°F or 65-75°C) using an oven.
- If using a dehydrator, preheat it according to the manufacturer's instructions.

How to Prepare the beef for drying:

- Remove the marinated beef from the refrigerator and discard any excess marinade.

- Pat beef slices dry with paper towels to remove excess moisture.

Drying of the beef:

- Arrange the beef slices in a single layer on a baking sheet (if using an oven) or on a rack set over a dehydrator tray.

- Using an oven, use a wooden spoon to open the oven door slightly to allow air to circulate.

- Dry the beef in the preheated oven or dehydrator until it is firm and dry.

- Depending on thickness and chewiness, it will take about 4-6 hours.

Store refrigerated:

- When the beef jerky is ready, please remove it from the oven or dehydrator and let it cool completely.
- Wipe the beef jerky dry with paper towels to remove any oil from the surface.

Beef jerky can be stored at room temperature for 1 to 2 weeks in an airtight or resealable bag. To store it for a long time, refrigerate or freeze the beef jerky.

You are enjoying homemade beef jerky as a delicious, protein-rich snack. Perfect for when you're traveling or need a hearty, carnivorous snack. Adjust seasonings to suit your taste preferences and experiment with different cuts of beef.

Bacon Stuffed Eggs

Ingredients:

- Six boiled eggs (peeled and cut in half lengthwise).
- Three slices of bacon, cooked until crispy and crumbly.
- Two tablespoons mayonnaise.
- One teaspoon of Dijon mustard.
- Salt and pepper for taste.
- Optional: paprika or minced garlic for garnish.

Instructions:

- Prepare the eggs.

- Cut boiled eggs in half lengthwise. Carefully remove the egg yolks and place them in a blender bowl.

- Place the egg whites cut in half on a plate.

Preparing the stuffing:

- Mash the egg yolks with a fork until smooth and crumbly.

- Add mayonnaise, Dijon mustard, and crumbled bacon to the egg yolk puree.

- Stir until smooth. Add salt and pepper to taste.

Egg white topping:

- Pour or squeeze the egg yolk mixture over the scooped white halves and distribute it evenly between them.

Garnish:

- If desired, sprinkle deviled eggs with paprika or minced garlic for added flavor and presentation.

Serve:

- Please put it on the Plate and serve immediately, or refrigerate until ready to eat.
- Enjoy our hearty and delicious bacon-deviled eggs as an appetizer or appetizer.

These bacon-deviled eggs will surely be a hit at any party or celebration. The combination of creamy egg yolks, savory bacon, and tangy mustard creates an explosion of flavor that's hard to resist.

Parmesan Cheese Chips

Ingredients to use in Making Parmesan Cheese Chips:

- One cup of freshly grated Parmesan cheese

Instructions:

Preheat oven: Preheat oven to 400°F (200°C).

Line a baking sheet with Foil paper or a silicone baking mat.

Forming of the Crips or Chips:

- Place small mounds (1 tablespoon each) of grated Parmesan cheese on the prepared baking sheet.
- Leave space in between to allow them to spread during baking.
- Lightly smooth out the mounds with the back of a spoon.

Baking of the Crisps:

- Transfer the baking sheet to the preheated oven and bake the Parmesan mounds for 3 to 5 minutes or until golden brown and crispy on the edges. Be careful, as it can burn quickly.

Allow to Cool and serve:

- Remove the baking sheet from the oven and let the Parmesan shavings cool on the baking sheet for a few minutes.

- Once the Parmesan shavings have cooled and solidified, carefully transfer them to a rack to cool completely and drain off any excess oil.

Serve Parmesan chips with a crunchy, delicious snack or appetizer. Enjoy on its own or combine with sauces, spreads, and salads for added texture and flavor. These parmesan chips are easy to make and incredibly delicious. He can create a crunchy, flavorful snack with just one ingredient, perfect for any occasion. Enjoy the exquisite combination of nutty Parmesan cheese and crunchy texture.

Chapter 9

Dessert (yes, even People on a carnivore diet can enjoy it!)

Bacon Chocolate Crust

Ingredients to use:

- Six pieces bacon
- 10 ounces of chopped dark chocolate (at least 70% cacao)
- 1/4 cup chopped nuts (such as almonds or pecans) (optional)
- Flaked sea salt for taste and sprinkling (optional)

Instructions on how to make:

Preparation of the bacon:

- Preheat oven to 400°F (200°C).

- Place bacon strips on a baking sheet lined with foil paper.

- Bake the bacon in the oven for 15 to 20 minutes or until crispy.

- Remove from the oven and transfer the bacon slices to a plate lined with paper towels to drain excess oil.

- Let cool completely, and then cut into small pieces.

Melting of the chocolate:

- Melt the chopped dark chocolate in a heatproof bowl set over a pot of boiling water (double boiler), stirring occasionally until smooth and completely melted.

- You can also melt the chocolate in the microwave a little at a time, stirring every 20 to 30 seconds until melted.

Preparing the bark:

- Line the baking line with parchment paper.
- Pour the melted chocolate onto the prepared baking sheet and spread it into an even layer with a spatula.

Add bacon and nuts:

- Sprinkle melted chocolate evenly over chopped bacon.
- If using chopped nuts, sprinkle them over the bacon.

Attach the bark

Place the mold in the refrigerator for about 1 hour or until the chocolate is formed.

Break it down into parts.

- When the chocolate dough is wholly hardened, please remove it from the refrigerator.
- Use your hands or a knife to break up the bark into pieces of the desired size.

Optional: Sprinkle with sea salt:

For an extra kick of flavor, sprinkle the chocolate crust pieces with flaky sea salt.

Serve and enjoy:

Arrange bacon chocolate chips on a plate or airtight container.

This Chocolate Bacon Crust combines dark chocolate's rich, indulgent flavor with the salty crunch of bacon to create a unique and delicious dessert that will impress. Enjoy as a special treat or gift to friends and family who appreciate the perfect balance of sweet and savory.

Creamy Cheesecake Bomb

Ingredients to use:

- 8 ounces cream cheese (softened)
- Four tablespoons softened unsalted butter
- 1/4 cup powdered erythritol or your favorite low-carb sweetener

- One teaspoon of vanilla extract

- Optional: lemon zest or extract for flavor.

- Optional toppings: unsweetened cocoa powder, chopped nuts, shredded coconut.

Instructions on how to make:

Mix the ingredients:

- Combine softened cream cheese and softened butter in a bowl. Mix until smooth and creamy. Add sweetness and flavor:

- Add powdered erythritol (your favorite sweetener) and vanilla extract to the cream cheese mixture. Mix well until thoroughly combined. Taste and adjust sweetness if necessary.

- If you like, add lemon zest or extract for a refreshing taste.

How to form a giant bomb:

- Use a spoon or cookie scoop to form the mixture into small balls and place on a baking sheet lined with parchment paper.

- You can also use silicone molds to make different shapes.

- If the mixture is too soft to handle, refrigerate briefly to firm up before shaping.

Coating (optional):

- Roll each giant bomb in unsweetened cocoa powder, chopped nuts, or shredded coconut for added texture and flavor.

- This step is optional but can add variety to your big bombs.

Refrigerating: Place the large, formed bombs in the refrigerator for at least 1 to 2 hours or until solidified.

Serving and storing:

- Once the large bombs have cooled and solidified, remove them from the refrigerator and place them in an airtight container.
- Serve chilled as a starter or hearty dessert. Leftovers can be stored in the refrigerator for up to 1 week.

Enjoy this oversized, creamy cheesecake bomb as a delicious and satisfying snack during your carnivore diet. Rich in healthy fats and low in carbohydrates, it's the perfect snack to energize and satisfy throughout the day. Customize the flavor and coating to suit your tastes and enjoy without feeling guilty!

Frozen steak (just kidding!)

Ahaha! Frozen steak slices may not be the most delicious idea, but it's always fun to experiment with culinary concepts. If you're interested in authentic carnivore-friendly recipes, let me know. We will be happy to provide it to you.

Chapter 10

Drinks

Homemade Bone Broth

Ingredients to use:

- 2 to 3 pounds of mixed bones (beef bones, chicken carcasses, pork bones, etc.)
- One onion, cut into quarters
- Two carrots (chopped)
- Two stalks of celery (chopped)
- Four cloves of garlic (chopped)
- Two bay leaves
- One tablespoon of apple cider vinegar
- Enough water to cover the bones
- Salt and pepper to taste (optional)

Instructions:

Roasting the bones you choose (optional):

- Preheat oven to 400°F (200°C).

- Place the bones on a baking sheet and roast in the oven for 30-45 minutes or until lightly browned and caramelized.

- This step is optional but adds depth to the soup's flavor.

We are preparing the soup in a pot.

- Transfer roasted bones (if using) to a large pot. Add onion, carrot, celery, garlic, bay leaf, and apple cider vinegar.

Filling the roasted bone with water:

- Fill the pot with enough water to cover the bones and vegetables by a few inches.

Cooking of the soup:

- Bring the water to a boil over high heat, then reduce the heat.
- Simmer the soup gently, uncovered, for at least 6 to 8 hours and up to 24 hours for maximum flavor.
- Remove any foam or debris that rose to the surface during cooking.

Straining the soup:

- Once the soup has boiled for the required time, please remove it from the stove.

- Using a fine sieve or cheesecloth, strain the soup into a clean pot or container, discarding the bones and vegetables.

Season (optional):

- Taste the soup and season with salt and pepper as needed.

- You can also customize the taste by adding other herbs and spices.

Storing in refrigeration:

- Let the soup cool to room temperature, then refrigerate overnight. This will allow the excess grease to solidify on the surface, making removing it easier.

- Remove any solidified fat from the surface of the soup and discard.

- Transfer the bone broth to an airtight container or freezer bag and store it in the refrigerator for up to 5 days or in the freezer for up to 6 months.

If desired, you can reheat bone broth and enjoy it as a nutritious and flavorful drink or as a base for soups, stews, sauces, and other dishes. Homemade bone broth is delicious and rich in collagen, minerals, and other beneficial compounds, making it incredibly nutritious.

Herbal Infusion

Ingredients to make use of:

- Fresh or dried herbs of your choice (mint, basil, rosemary, Thyme, lavender, etc.)
- Water
- Optional: Sweetener (such as honey or stevia).

Instructions:

Choosing an herb: Select the herbs to use for the infusion. You can create your flavor profile using a single herb or a combination of different herbs.

Preparing the herbs:

If using fresh herbs, rinse them under cold water to remove dirt and debris. If using dried herbs, measure out the amount you need.

Heating of water for the herbs:

Boil the water in a pot or kettle. The water you use depends on how strong you want the infusion and how much you plan on making.

Infuse herbs:

- Once the water boils, please remove it from the heat and add fresh or dried herbs to the pot or kettle.
- Cover the pot or kettle and steep the herbs in boiling water for 5 to 10 minutes or until the desired flavor is achieved.

- Steeping time will vary depending on the herbs used and personal preference.

Filtering of the infusion solution:

- After steeping, filter the decoction to remove the herbs.
- For this step, you can use a fine mesh strainer, cheesecloth, or tea infuser.

Sweeten (optional):

- If desired, sweeten the infusion with honey, stevia, or another sweetener, and avoid using artificial sweeteners.
- Stir until the sweetener is completely dissolved.

Serve and enjoy:

- Pour the infusion into a cup or mug and serve warm.

- Cool to room temperature and add ice to create a refreshing frozen herbal drink.

Herbal infusions are a delicious way to enjoy herbs' natural flavors and benefits. Experiment with different herb combinations and adjust the infusion time to your preference. Herbal infusions are calming and energizing drinks that can be enjoyed hot or cold at any time of the day.

Coffee and Tea tips for Carnivores Diet

Here are some tips for meat eaters who want to follow their dietary preferences and enjoy coffee and tea.

Coffee

Black Coffee Option: Enjoy black coffee without added sugar, milk, or cream. Black coffee is naturally low in calories and carbohydrates, making it suitable for carnivore diets.

Choose high-quality beans

Look for high-quality, freshly roasted coffee beans. Experiment with different roasts and origins to find your favorite flavor.

Avoid flavored coffee

Avoid flavored coffee beans and syrups, as they often contain added sugars and artificial flavors incompatible with a carnivore's diet.

Monitor your intake

Although coffee is generally considered safe in moderation, excessive caffeine intake can cause harmful side effects such as nervousness, anxiety, and sleep problems. Listen to your body and adjust your coffee intake accordingly.

Tea

Keep your tea simple. Choose simple, unsweetened teas such as black, green, white, or herbal. Avoid flavored teas that have added sugar or artificial flavors.

Try herbal tea: Herbal teas, also called infusions, are made from various herbs, flowers, and spices. They are caffeine-free and provide a pleasant, flavorful alternative to traditional caffeinated teas.

Consider infusing bone broth.: Add some warm bone broth to your tea to enhance its effect. This creates a unique flavor profile and adds extra nutrients and vitamins to your drink.

Be careful with herbal blends: Some herbal tea blends may contain ingredients incompatible with a carnivore's diet, such as fruits, grains, and seeds. Read the ingredient list carefully, or use single-ingredient herbal teas to meet your dietary preferences.

Be careful in choosing herbs: Many herbal teas are suitable for carnivorous diets, while others have laxative and diuretic properties. Pay attention to your body's response to herbal teas and adjust your intake accordingly.

It can be served hot or cold, depending on your preference and the weather. Experiment with different brewing methods and serving temperatures to find what you like best.

By following these tips, carnivores can continue enjoying their coffee or tea while achieving their dietary goals. Whether you're drinking hot black coffee or enjoying soothing herbal tea, countless options suit every taste and occasion.

Chapter 11

Tips for Meal Planning and Success

Weekly Meal Planning Guide for People Aiming to Follow a Carnivore Diet

Note. This meal plan is a general guide. Adjust portion sizes and ingredients based on your needs, preferences, and dietary goals.

Day one

Breakfast

Scrambled eggs fried in butter

Bacon Slices

Lunch

Grilled Chicken Thighs

Beef Bone Broth

Ribeye Steak

Sautéed spinach with garlic and olive oil.

Day two

Sausage patties

Fried eggs

Tuna salad (canned tuna mixed with chopped pickles and mayonnaise)

Beef bone broth

Pork chops

Steamed broccoli with some butter

Day Three

Steak and eggs (Preferably fried with butter)

Bacon strips

Grounded beef made with onions and spices

Beef bone broth

Lamb chops

Creamed spinach (cooked spinach mixed with Parmesan cheese and cream)

Day Four

Breakfast

Bacon-wrapped sausages

Scrambled eggs are preferably cooked in bacon fat.

Lunch

Grilled salmon fillets

Beef bone broth

Dinner

Liver (Assorted beef) cooked in butter

Caesar salad (romaine lettuce, Caesar dressing and Parmesan cheese)

Day Five

Breakfast

Chicken liver

Fried eggs

Lunch

Grounded beef burger patties

Beef bone broth

Dinner

Pan-seared duck breasts

Asparagus spears: Preferably cooked in bacon fat.

Day Six

Breakfast

Egg muffins (eggs baked with bacon or sausage)

Lunch

Grilled shrimp skewers

Beef bone broth

Dinner

Beef short ribs cooked in bone broth

Creamy cauliflower mash

Day Seven

Breakfast

Bacon and cheese omelet

Lunch

Beef brisket slices

Beef bone broth

Dinner

Grilled lamb kebabs

Roasted Brussels sprouts with bacon

Snacks (optional)

Cheese slice

Pork skin

Beef Jerky

Boiled egg

SOME TIPS FOR BEGINNERS

During the day, drink water or bone soup to maintain hydration and replenish electrolytes.

Experiment with various meats, cooking methods, and seasonings to make your dishes exciting and comfortable. Listen to your body and adjust your portion sizes and meal ration based on your hunger and energy needs.

Consult your health care professional or dietitian before starting a new diet, especially if you have any health conditions or dietary restrictions. A carnivore diet makes dinner both enjoyable and satisfying. Here are some tips for navigating restaurant menus while maintaining your nutritional preferences.

Choose a steakhouse or barbecue restaurant.

Steakhouses and barbecue restaurants often offer a variety of perfectly cooked meat dishes. Look for steaks like ribeye, sirloin, filet mignon, barbecue ribs, brisket, smoked meats, and more.

Choose simple preparation.

Use simple, lightly seasoned, or marinated meats to avoid added sugars and carbohydrates. Grilled, fried, or baked meats are generally safe choices.

Request personal customization.

Don't hesitate to ask your server to make changes based on your dietary needs. Order a steak cooked without oil or marinade and ask to substitute meat or bacon for vegetables or garnishes.

Choose protein-rich snacks.

Start your meal with protein-rich appetizers like shrimp cocktail, oysters on the half shell, and beef tartare. These options are generally low in carbohydrates and pair well with carnivore diets.

Be careful with sauces and dressings.

Be wary of sauces, dressings, and condiments containing added sugars or ingredients unsuitable for carnivore diets. Ask for more sauce or omit it entirely.

Check out the side dish options.

Many restaurant side dishes are high in carbohydrates, but some may offer carnivore-friendly options, such as sautéed spinach, creamed spinach, or steamed broccoli.

Consider fasting or eating before.

If you're unsure of the options or want to stick to meat, consider fasting or snacking before eating out. This way, you can focus on the social aspects of dinner without compromising your dietary goals.

Stay hydrated.

Drink plenty of water or sugar-free drinks to stay hydrated and avoid feeling hungry or hungry during meals.

Practice mindful eating

Take your time and savor each bite of your food. Concentrate on the taste and texture of the meat and listen to your body's hunger and satiety signals.

Enjoy the experience.

Eating out is as much about the experience as the food. Relax, enjoy the company of your peers, and enjoy the opportunity to explore different cuisines while living a carnivorous lifestyle. By following these tips, you can eat confidently, continue your journey on the Carnivore diet, and enjoy delicious, satisfying meals while adhering to your dietary preferences.

Troubleshooting Common Issues

Switching to a carnivore diet can present many challenges for beginners. Here are some common issues and troubleshooting tips to overcome them.

Symptoms of carbohydrate withdrawal:

Problem: When switching to a carnivore diet, some people experience carbohydrate withdrawal symptoms such as fatigue, headaches, irritability, and cravings.

Troubleshooting: Be patient and give your body time to adjust to the new diet. Stay hydrated, prioritize your intake of electrolytes (sodium, potassium, and magnesium), and consider reducing your carbohydrate intake gradually rather than suddenly.

Digestive problems:

Problem: As your body adapts to increased meat and fat intake, you may experience digestive issues such as constipation and diarrhea.

Solution: Increase your water intake, incorporate bone broth to support gut health, and gradually increase your intake of fatty meats to help your digestive system adjust. Consider incorporating fermented foods like sauerkraut and kimchi to encourage the growth of beneficial gut bacteria.

Social pressure and prejudice:

The challenge: Dealing with social pressure and prejudice from friends, family, and colleagues who may not understand or support your decision to follow a carnivore diet.

Troubleshooting: Learn the benefits of the carnivore diet and be prepared to explain your food choices to others. Surround yourself with supportive people who respect your decisions and focus on the positive aspects of your dietary journey.

Variety and boredom:

Problem: Feeling bored or restricted by the carnivore diet, especially the lack of variety in food options.

Troubleshoot: Add variety to your dishes by changing cooking methods, seasonings, and cuts of meat. Try different types of animal proteins, organs, and seafood. Find carnivore-friendly recipes and meal ideas to keep your meals exciting and fun.

Nutritional deficiencies:

Challenges: Concerns about potential nutritional deficiencies, especially vitamins, minerals, and fiber, when following a carnivore diet.

Troubleshooting: Focus on eating a variety of animal proteins, including lean meats, poultry, fish, and organ meats, to ensure you're getting a wide range of nutrients. Consider incorporating nutrient-rich foods into your diet, such as bone broth, eggs, and liver. Monitor your energy levels, mood, and overall health, and consult your doctor if you have concerns about your nutrient intake.

Cravings and emotional eating:

The challenge: managing the cravings and emotional triggers that can arise when adopting a carnivore diet.

Troubleshoot: Practice mindful eating and listen to your body's hunger and satiety signals. Find other ways to deal with stress and emotional triggers, such as practicing relaxation techniques, walking, or pursuing a hobby. Focus on the long-term benefits of a carnivore diet and stay true to your health goals.

By addressing these common issues and implementing troubleshooting strategies, beginners can transition to a carnivore diet more quickly and confidently. Remember, everyone's carnivore diet experience is different. Be patient with yourself and listen to your body as you embark on this weight loss journey.

Conclusion

Conclusion: Adopting a carnivorous lifestyle

Starting your carnivore diet journey as a beginner can be exciting and challenging. As you've learned in this guide, switching to a diet focused primarily on animal products has many potential benefits, including better weight management, increased energy levels, and improved overall health. However, it is essential to approach this diet with awareness, knowledge, and a willingness to adapt.